Table of Contents

Table of Contents

Introduction

Keep up to Date with New Releases

Chapter 1 What is Snoring?

Chapter 2 Typical Causes of Snoring

Chapter 3 Snoring due to Underlying Health Conditions

Chapter 4 Finding the Right Cure

Chapter 5 Traditional Home Snoring Remedies

Chapter 6 Medical Cures for Snoring

Steps to Success Action Plan

Conclusion

Other Books you may be interested in...

Free Gift

Introduction

Are you worried you'll never have a good night sleep again?

Do you struggle in your daily life because you're tired from being up all night snoring, or listening to a loved one snore?

Is snoring starting to affect your personal life? You're Relationship?

Are you starting to worry about your health because of snoring?

Do you wish you knew how to treat snoring once and for all?

Or are you just plain sick of being hit by your partner all night?

In this book you will discover the most up-to-date information on snoring, and the best ways to treat it including:

-Why people actually snore

-What causes people to snore?

-What the different types of snoring are

-How to find the right cure for you!

And much more!

I want to thank you and congratulate you for downloading the book, Stop Snoring Today; Practical techniques to stop you snoring once and for all!

My name is Simone, and I am the creator of the Healthy Body Books. I would like to take this opportunity to tell you who I am and why I decided to create this helpful tool.

My passion for health extends beyond the superficial. A part of me has always been called to make health a priority in my life. I am dedicated to making my body perfect, at least the way I see it.

Unfortunately, one change in my routine made it that much harder to obtain the perfect body. I found myself not feeling as good as I used to, and I even felt like I could not longer achieve my goals. To put it bluntly, I was concerned for my health and my future.

After searching long and hard for potential solutions to my problem, I found relief in changing my diet, natural therapies and self-help. Using a number of natural techniques, I was finally able to get my life back under control – and it felt great! I felt like things were really the way they were supposed to be.

If you are trying to find another way to stay healthy, the Healthy Body Books are meant for you. If you feel like something in your life just isn't working and might even be stopping you from living the life you want to live, you will find solace in new techniques and knowledge. Each book is written by experts, but the everyday person will be able to read and the books with ease.

Good luck!

Snoring can be a debilitating condition that can really control your life. In this book you will find the most up-to-date information on how to get rid of that pesky and bothersome snoring and save your relationship with your bedmate from falling apart.

Good Luck

Keep up to Date with New Releases

Thank you again for downloading this Kindle Book Stop Snoring Today; Practical techniques to stop you snoring once and for all!

I'd like to offer you the chance to stay up-to date on new books with free access to my newsletter!

You will be getting up to date information on health, fitness and diet, and also get access to getting other Healthy Body Books for free. By joining my newsletter you will be taking a big step forward in being your Healthiest Body yet!

Just visit http://www.healthybodybooks.com and get free instant access to the Healthy Body Books newsletter today!

Chapter 1 What is Snoring?

Snoring is that loud often-irritating sound produced when respiratory tissues block the air passage and start to vibrate as the person breathes in air while sleeping. It is a condition that is considered commonplace especially since 45% of the male population and approximately a third of females snore regularly while asleep.

The funny part is people who snore never really realizes they do until somebody tells them so. They are too deep in their sleep to know they are snoring. And, when someone informs them about it, they are even likely to treat the information with a grain of salt.

The most concerning thing about snoring is the fact that people who snore are totally oblivious of it. They are too deep in their sleep to be bothered by it. Snoring is more of a problem of the bedmates or the people sleeping near or around those who snore. The noise they create can be so irritating and bothersome that others are likely to lose sleep over them.

Snoring does not ordinarily pose a serious health risk except for some that are caused by underlying health conditions, which we will be discussing in a separate chapter. Otherwise it is quite commonplace. Consider these statistics based on a survey made by Vancouver Sleep and Breathing Center as verified on July 28, 2013:

30% of the population aged 30 and above snores;

40%of the population aged 40 and above snores;

19% of the female population snores;

5.6% of the children population snores;

59% of those surveyed say their bed partners snores.

On the average, snoring produces at least 38 decibels, which would be like sleeping right next to a humming refrigerator or a running dishwasher. Never the less, snoring is quite commonplace if we base it on its prevalence as gleaned from the above statistics.

But no matter how commonplace snoring may be, it surely can ruin relationships or even break up marriages. The fact is snoring is the number 3 cause for divorce - just slightly behind financial problems and infidelity. It is also the number one medical reason for most of the divorce cases filed on 2013. If you want to save a relationship marred by the bothersome snoring of a partner, or if you simply want to put a stop to the snoring of your bedmate, then what you need to do is to identify the cause of the snoring first (there are a number of them) before you can put in place the most appropriate and the most effective remedy.

There is no single 'cure-all' shotgun remedy for snoring. You need to first identify the real cause of the snoring before you consider what course of action to take. Besides, as mentioned earlier, there are people who snore because of some serious underlying health conditions, which should never be ignored. This e-book contains a lot of invaluable information about snoring as well as a host of tried and tested remedies to cure people of their snoring.

Chapter 2 Typical Causes of Snoring

Essentially, snoring is the result of narrowed nasal air passage. We naturally breathe through the nose and rarely from the mouth. When we breathe we let air flow in and out from the nose (or in some instances from the mouth) to the lungs. Our bodies prefer to breathe air through the nose since the nasal cavities actually filter and clean the air we breathe.

Sometimes, however, obstructions can occur in the nasal airways where the air passes to and from the lungs. This results in a narrowed air passage, which in turn creates turbulence in the airflow. The turbulence in the airflow causes the tissues in the nasal cavity to vibrate producing sound waves, which we commonly refer to as snoring.

The Soft Palate and the Uvula

Normally, it is the soft palate and the small extension at the back of the soft palate called the uvula, which usually blocks the airflow and produces the snoring sounds. The soft palate is a muscular extension of the roof of the mouth. Together with the uvula, they help in swallowing food and directing it to the stomach. They also help to channel the air we breathe through the pharynx into our lungs. When on a resting mode particularly when we are sleeping, the soft palate and/or the uvula can collapse and form an obstruction to the flow of air we breathe.

This is how it happens. When we go to sleep, the brain sends signals to every muscle tissue of the body to relax and stop working - except of course those muscles needed for breathing. The soft palate and the nebula are among those that collapse into a relaxed mode when we fall asleep.

If either the soft palate or uvula happens to be too long, it may somewhat narrow the air passage and somehow block the airflow once it collapses when it goes into a relax mode. This creates the turbulence, which causes these tissues to vibrate and produce the snoring sound.

The Nasal Turbinate's

The nose also has what are referred to as the nasal turbinate's. These are cylindrical passages lying parallel to the nasal floor cavity. They help regulate the flow of air through the nose. The turbinate's contained blood vessels, which make them swell (increase in size) or constrict (become narrower). When more blood is pumped to the blood vessels in the turbinate's, the blood vessels become enlarged making the turbinate's also swell in size thus decreasing the flow of air passing through them.

When the blood that goes into these blood vessels lessens, the blood vessels start to constrict. When this happens, the turbinate's also become smaller allowing more air to pass through.

The nasal turbinate's naturally cycles through these phases alternately and on a regular basis every day. However, the turbinate's can remain swollen far longer than normal during certain instances like when you catch cold or have a stuffy nose due to allergic reactions to dirt or cold air. This leaves the person with no option but to breathe air through the mouth.

With obstruction in the nasal airway people will have to breathe through their mouths. But, breathing air through the mouth actually causes greater and more vigorous vibrations of the nasal tissues. This is basically the reason why most of those who breathe air through their mouths when they sleep normally end up snoring.

The Tonsils and Adenoids

Among children, tonsillitis and infection of the adenoid (the tonsils located at the back of the throat) are often the cause of the narrowed nasal air passage. The main role of the tonsils is to block infection.

The tonsils become enlarged when they are fighting infections. Unfortunately, they tend to remain enlarged even after the infection is gone. The now enlarged tonsils or adenoids eventually narrow the air passage which in turn results into snoring.

Among adults, narrowed air passages may also result from sinus infections, allergies, or septal deviations.

The Tongue

The tongue plays an important role of properly directing and managing the food we eat as we chew and swallow them but they also can block air passage when it collapses into a resting mode.

The tongue has to be flexible enough to be able to move in any direction for it to do the job of directing food more efficiently. This is why it is not rigidly fixed at the tip or at the top. And since it is not rigidly fixed in one place, it has the tendency to slide too far back when we are asleep thus narrowing the air passage through the pharynx into the lungs. At times too, the tongue happens to be too large or too thick such that the back of the tongue creates a narrower air passage through the pharynx. This produces greater and more turbulent vibrations in the nasal tissues as we suck in air through the mouth eventually producing more disturbing snoring sounds.

Medications and alcohol

Alcohol and some medications enhance the relaxation of your muscles when you sleep. As a result, the palate, uvula, neck, tongue, and pharynx collapses totally causing a blockade of the nasal airways and further narrowing the air passage. This worsens snoring even more.

Sleep Posture

Gravity tends to pull your muscles down when you are sleeping. If you sleep flat on your back the tongue, the palate, and the muscles of your throat to relax. Gravity pulls them down further making them block the airway passages and making you snore in the process. Rolling over to your side unblocks the airways and stops the snoring.

Aging

When people reach middle age and over, the muscle tone in the throat and the tongue slackens. The throat becomes narrower and the tongue tends to slide back a bit further creating a narrowed air passage. The narrowed airway passage causes you to snore.

Too Much Fatty Tissue in the throat

Being obese or overweight can mean having a bulky throat that is enwrapped in fatty tissues. The fatty tissues surrounding the throat actually squeezes the throat making the airway passage narrower thereby causing the snore. The floppy fat tissues around the throat are also prone to vibrate and worsen the snoring.

Primary Snoring does not really pose a Serious Health Risk

All of the snore factors discussed above are the primary causes of snoring and are totally unrelated to any underlying health condition. Which means a healthy person may snore yet he breathes normally while asleep. He is in no danger to any health risk.

However, not all snoring is the same. It is important that you are able to differentiate between primary snoring (those that are caused by the various factors discussed above and the snoring which results from an underlying health condition such as what we will be discussing in the next chapter.

Chapter 3 Snoring due to Underlying Health Conditions

Snoring can be a manifestation of an underlying health condition. More specifically, it may indicate that the person may be suffering from a condition called sleep apnea a sleep disorder where breathing abnormally pauses for ten to seconds for several times during sleep.

What happens during each sleep apnea episode is the airflow completely stops briefly and the oxygen level in the blood starts to drop. The brain responds by jolting you enough out of your sleep and kick start your breathing once more. Breathing resumes with a choking or gasping sound. You are briefly awakened to tighten up the throat muscles and open the air passage once more. However, you will hardly remember these brief episodes as you normally go back to sleep again. These sleep apnea episodes can occur up to a hundred times in a single night and you won't even remember any of it.

There are three types of sleep apneas – the most common type is known as the Obstructive Sleep Apnea (OSA), the less common Central Sleep Apnea (CSA), and the Complex Sleep Apnea, which is a combination of the first and the second. With the Obstructive Sleep Apnea, the soft tissues at the back of the throat relaxes when you fall asleep and totally collapses to block the airway passage producing a loud snoring sound in the process. With Central Sleep apnea, the apnea episodes occur because the brain fails to transmit signals to the muscles that control breathing.

People suffering from sleep apnea are not really aware that they have this difficulty in breathing. They could hardly remember the brief apnea episodes no matter how many times they occur in a single night. They will just feel fatigued the whole day feeling drowsy and sleepy most of the time. Often, it is the bed partner or anyone who happens to sleep in the same room that notices the difficulty in his breathing.

It is difficult to identify sleep apnea on your own. You will need professional assistance to be able to do it. However, it will help a lot if you can get your partner to help you observe the common symptoms of this sleep disorder. Among the symptoms are:

Abnormally long pauses (10 to 20 seconds) in breathing while asleep.

Exceptionally loud and chronic snoring no matter what sleeping posture is.

Frequent gasping, choking, or snorting during sleep.

Daytime Drowsiness despite having long hours of sleep.

Left untreated, sleep apnea can be a potentially dangerous disorder. More than half of those with sleep apnea are hypertensive while about half of those with essential hypertension have sleep apnea. They have 4x more chances of having a stroke and 3x more chances of acquiring a heart condition.

According to the latest statistics, one out of 15 American adults has sleep apnea while up to 10% of children can be afflicted by it. The best thing to do is to immediately see your doctor once you spot any of the symptoms we've mentioned above. The difficulty of determining whether you have sleep apnea stems from the fact that not everyone who snores has sleep apnea and not everyone with sleep apnea snores. It is best to consult your doctor immediately at the onset of the warning signs.

Chapter 4 Finding the Right Cure

Remember that before you can find the cure you must first identify the cause and the remedy you choose must be the one that addresses the cause of the snoring right on the head. At this point it will help a lot if you observe a person's sleep posture and how he snores. The sleep posture and how he snores will give you a clue on what causes the snore. But you will need to get the help of your bed partner to help you jot down observations while you sleep on some sort of a sleep diary.

The entries made to your sleep diary will contain valuable information that can help make a self-diagnosis of your condition. And should you consult a doctor in the future your sleep diary will help the doctor a lot in making a more objective assessment of your snoring. He will know exactly how and where to proceed to correct the condition.

The entries on your sleep diary will reveal what exactly causes the snore. Armed with this knowledge, you should be able to find the most appropriate home remedy to stop the snoring.

Here are some helpful hints you can use to help you determine the cause of the snoring:

A person who snores while sleeping with his mouth closed indicates that the problem may lie in the tongue.

A person who snores while sleeping with an open mouth may indicate a problem in the tissues surrounding the throat.

If a person snores only while sleeping on his back indicates only a mild case of snoring, which can be corrected with some lifestyle changes, and improving the sleeping habits.

A person who snores in all sleep postures may indicate a more severe case of snoring, which will definitely require a more comprehensive remedy. It is best to seek professional help for this than attempt to correct the condition on your own.

The bottom line is there are really no known cures that will totally eliminate snoring. At best, what you will encounter are remedies meant to minimize snoring and bring it down to a tolerable level. You may be surprised to see tons upon tons of snore stop over-the-counter products being sold today but sadly most of them don't work. Those that work are just 50 to 60% effective. Even experts in the field of respiratory medicine are quite skeptical about these products. So, before you fall prey to the marketing innuendos of these over the counter products, try the traditional, proven home remedies to stop snoring first.

Start by introducing some vital changes to your lifestyle - paying particular attention to the things that aggravate snoring like:

Losing weight if you happen to be quite a bit heavy on all sides. Losing weight will reduce the floppy fat tissues at the back of your throat, which usually block or narrow the airway passage. This will help decrease if not totally eliminate snoring.

Engage in regular exercises. Exercise will not only strengthen your arms, abs, and legs, it will also improve the muscle tone of the tissues around the throat so that when you sleep these tissues will not totally collapse and form a blockade to your airway passage.

If you are a regular smoker, it is high time that you quit. Smoking blocks the nasal airways in case you are not aware of it.

Avoid taking alcohol or any sleep inducing medication before bedtime. They will make you fall into a deeper sleep and relax your mouth, throat, and nose muscles more to a point that they block the nasal air passage.

Change your diet. It is a known fact that the kind of food we eat has a great impact on our body functions. It has also been proven time and again that a Ketogenic diet, which is low in carbohydrates, high fat, and with adequate protein, can minimize if not totally eliminate snoring.

Avoid taking simple sugars such as sweets and soft drinks before bedtime. Simple sugars cause mild dehydration, which forces our body to breathe through the mouth instead of the nose. Needless to say, mouth breathers usually snore.

Chapter 5 Traditional Home Snoring Remedies

There are many tried and tested home remedies that have been proven to be effective in minimizing if not totally eliminating snoring. They are inexpensive yet more effective than commercial snore stop products, which have been crowding the supermarket shelves, and bombarding the airwaves with advertising. So before you spend a fortune on these products give them a try first.

Make it a point to sleep with your head elevated. This way pressure is taken away from the nasal airway allowing you to breathe easier. Don't just raise your head by stuffing more pillows under it. This will squeeze and narrow the airways more aggravating the situation. Instead, elevate the head of the bed by putting blocks of wood under the posts. It is important that you prop up the whole upper body and not just the head.

Make sure the bedroom air is moist and not dry. Dry air irritates the nasal and throat membranes making them swell and narrow the air passage as a result. Use a humidifier or a steam vaporizer to do this.

Avoid heavy meals, soymilk, dairy products and caffeine a couple of hours before bedtime.

Avoid sleeping lying flat on your back and sleep on your side instead. If you can't get used to sleeping on your side you can try the old 'tennis ball trick. Sew a sock to the back of your pajamas and insert a tennis ball in it. Every time you try laying on your back the tennis ball will stop you from doing it and force you to sleep on your side instead. After some time, you will feel comfortable sleeping on your side and you won't have a need for the tennis ball again.

Before bedtime, take a couple of sips of olive oil. This trick has been proven over and over again to lessen snoring.

Alternately, you can try to gargle with sage extracts before going to bed. Put a handful of sage in a pot of boiling water and allow it to steep. Let it cool and strain the mixture. Gargle with the liquid.

You can also try gargling with a peppermint mouthwash before going to bed. This will shrink the linings of your mouth and nose. This has been proven to be extremely effective in cases where snoring is due to colds or allergy.

If your nasal cavities are clogged up due to allergy or colds you can try unclogging them using a bowl of boiling water. Cover your head with a towel and bend over the bowl of boiling water with your nose barely 15 centimeters away from the bowl. Make sure to cover the bowl with your towel as well. Start breathing deeply through your nose and continue breathing for a few minutes.

Make sure you are well hydrated before going to bed. Drink enough water all throughout the day especially before bedtime. When you go to sleep a bit dehydrated, the body responds by forcing you to breathe through your mouth, which usually leads to snoring.

Try to exercise your tongue regularly before bedtime. There are tongue exercises you can do to strengthen the tongue and prevent it from falling and blocking the airways when you fall asleep. Try making the sound like "ta-ta-ta-ta-ta" as if you are scolding someone. Repeat five times. This strengthens the tip of the tongue. To strengthen the sides of the tongue, stick your tongue out as far as you can and let it hang relaxed then point and hold it for three seconds. Repeat the exercise 10 times.

Try putting two drops of clarified butter in each nostril every night before going to bed and another two drops in the morning. Instead of clarified butter, you can use Brahmi oil (ayuverdic herbal oil), which you can easily get online.

Another home remedy alternative is to mix two teaspoons of turmeric powder with a glass of warm milk and consume it before bedtime.

You can also try some yoga breathing exercises like Pranayama. It has been used as a relaxation technique to relieve many sleep disorders like sleep apnea. Yoga exercises allow you to control your breathing and make you breathe easily even while you sleep.

Chapter 6 Medical Cures for Snoring

Don't lose hope if you've tried every home remedy you can lay your hands on and still the snoring persists. There are still the medical cures and treatments to turn to. If everything you've tried so far has failed, the best thing to do is see the doctor. This time around, you are more knowledgeable about your predicament. With the knowledge you've gained about snoring so far, you may have probably identified the cause of your snoring. This puts you in a vantage position to discuss your snoring problems with your doctor. And, if you've followed, every tip in this book, you must have your sleep diary ready with you. The diary can be truly helpful to your doctor in diagnosing your case. The valuable information contained therein will help him determine the most appropriate cure to eliminate your snoring once and for all with great ease.

Never be tempted to try the commercially available, over the counter snore stop products without seeing your doctor first. You can be ripped off by many of these OTC products that don't work. Go see your doctor first. But before you do, it is best that you also become familiar with most of the available medical cures and treatments to correct snoring. That way, when your doctor makes a recommendation, you will know exactly what he is talking about. Best of all, knowing the various medical cures available will prevent you from being ripped off by your own doctor since he'll be aware that you know what he is talking about.

Medical cures for snoring

Medical cures and treatment can be divided into two categories – the non-surgical and the surgical.

Non-Surgical Methods

The non-surgical medical treatments for snoring are essentially non-invasive and include the following:

Continuous Positive Airway Pressure Machine (CPAP). This device blows a continuous flow of pressurized air into a mask you wear on your face. Doctors normally prescribe this device to adults with sleep apnea.

Mandibular Repositioning Splints – These are dental appliances that resemble mouth guards to help keep your airways open. This device brings the lower jaw forward and prevents the tongue from relaxing backwards when you sleep.

Nasal devices such as nasal strips and nasal dilators meant to keep the nostrils always open when you sleep.

Vestibular shield that looks like a gum shield and used to prevent you from breathing through your mouth and force you to breathe through your nose instead.

Medications and sprays meant to correct inflammation due to infection or allergy. They are meant to shrink the nasal cavities and clear the airway passage.

Lifestyle changes such as those discussed in the previous chapters. Many of the snoring cases can be corrected with a simple lifestyle change the objective of which is to eliminate all and everything that may aggravate snoring from the food you eat to the way you sleep.

Surgical Methods

Surgical treatment for snoring is only done when the cause of the snoring have been verified beyond doubt. Such procedures are normally done on the nasal passages, tongue, palate and uvula and are totally irreversible that is why the need for prior verification.

The surgical procedures involves repair, scarring, implants, and removal of tissues most of which can be done in a doctor's office while the more sensitive ones like those requiring anesthesia have to be performed in the operating rooms. But before you decide to have surgical treatment to correct your snoring, you should check with your health insurance company to determine which procedures are covered as well as the estimated cost of surgery that is covered.

Some of these surgical procedures to correct snoring can actually be had for free from the National Health Services (NHS) as long as you can prove to them that your snoring is adversely affecting your quality of life as well as your over-all health and that you have tried without success all the other treatment options recommended by your doctor.

Please note that before any surgical procedure is done to correct the snoring you must undergo polysomnogram or a formal sleep study. This is to verify the cause of the snoring and to discount the possibility that snoring may be due to sleep apnea.

Proceeding with any surgical procedure to correct snoring without such a study may leave sleep apnea undiagnosed or undetected which can lead to a more serious condition later on because you'll just be eliminating the symptom without correcting the breathing problem. Besides, if the snoring is because of sleep apnea there is no need for a surgical procedure since the non-surgical CPAP procedure will suffice.

The surgical treatments to correct snoring include:

Traditional surgery such as tonsillectomy, adenoidectomy, Thermal Ablation Palatoplasty (TAP), and Uvulopalatopharyngoplasty (UPPP). These procedures are meant to clear and enlarge the airway passages by surgically removing the corresponding tissues or repairing certain abnormalities.

The Pillar procedure – This procedure is meant to strengthen the soft palate after it has been verified that it is the palate that is causing the snoring. The procedure involves inserting plastic implants into the soft palate. The implants will in time be wrapped with scar tissues stiffening it and preventing it from unnecessarily vibrating which causes the snoring.

Laser-assisted uvulopalatoplasty (LAUP) – This procedure uses laser to remove parts of an excessively long soft palate that is blocking the airway passage when you sleep. The surgery is usually done in a doctor's office and requires three to five visits with each visit lasting no more than 30 minutes. Please proceed with great caution on this since the AMA or American Medical Association is against the use of laser technology to performoperationson the uvula or on the pharynx.

Radiofrequency tissue ablation (somnoplasty) – This is another procedure that can be done in the doctor's office and like the LAUP, it is used to correct the snoring caused by an extra long soft palate. The difference is instead of cutting the palate it shrinks the tissues of the soft palate using radio frequency with low intensity settings. It is done under anesthesia and is less painful than other surgical procedures.

Uvulectomy - This is a simple procedure meant to remove the uvula after determining that it is the cause of snoring. It can be done at the doctor's office on a single visit. However, you need to prepare to handle two to three weeks of pain and discomfort after the procedure. You also run the risk of excessive bleeding and altered speech. If you speak Hebrew or Farsi or any other language that uses guttural fricatives (consonant sounds produced with the use of the uvula) then your speech may be severely impaired. This is of no consequence though to English speaking people since the English language does not have guttural fricatives.

Tongue Suspension Procedure – More popularly known as the Repose™ system, the procedure is meant to make the base of the tongue more stable to prevent it from falling back and blocking the airway passage when you fall asleep. It involves the use of a titanium screw, which is fixed to the lower jaw and attached to the base of the tongue with a suture. This is designed to hold the tongue forward instead of falling further back when you fall asleep. The system has the FDA approval since 1998. It can be done at the doctor's office and takes only about 15to 20 minutes to finish. This is a relatively new procedure that may require further assessment so proceed with caution.

Injection snoreplasty – This is a procedure to correct snoring due to a fluttering floppy uvula. It was developed by Army doctors at the Walter Reed Hospital in 2000. The procedure involves injecting a hardening agent (sodium tetradecyl sulfate) just under the skin in front of the uvula on the roof of the mouth. This will create a blister, which will harden into a scar tissue later on. The hardened scar tissue pulls the uvula forward preventing or minimizing its flutter and effectively reducing the snore. This procedure is 92% more effective than LAUP and is relatively safer.

Steps to Success Action Plan

Steps to Success have been put together to give you somewhere to start on getting rid of your snoring. Having a restful night's sleep is the goal, and by starting with the activities listed here you will be well on your way to a wonderful night's sleep in no time!

To really have success you may need to use this action plan a few times and trial a few different things to get the result you're after. Test, Measure and Monitor needs to become your motto until you are having undisturbed nights again.

Step 1- Read Chapter 1 to fully understand what is snoring

Step 2- Diagnose Causes of snoring that you may have

Step 3 -Decide what causes of snoring you can eliminate straight away

Step 4 –Test these out for 3 nights and see if they have the desired effect

Step 5- If the desired result has not been achieved please go back to causes of snoring and see if there is anything else you can eliminate. From here you need to start trying the home remedies. Pick 1 home remedy and try it for 3 nights.

Step 6- How did you go with trying a home remedy for 3 nights? Success? If not try another one of the home remedies for another 3 nights and see if that works.

Step 7- If you find you have tried all of the home remedies and nothing is working it might be time to look into medical cures for snoring. At this stage you will need to go and talk to your local GP about what options will suit you in moving forward.